Simple Keto Snacks

Reduce Your Hunger with These Tasty
Treats!

Table of Contents

Introduction

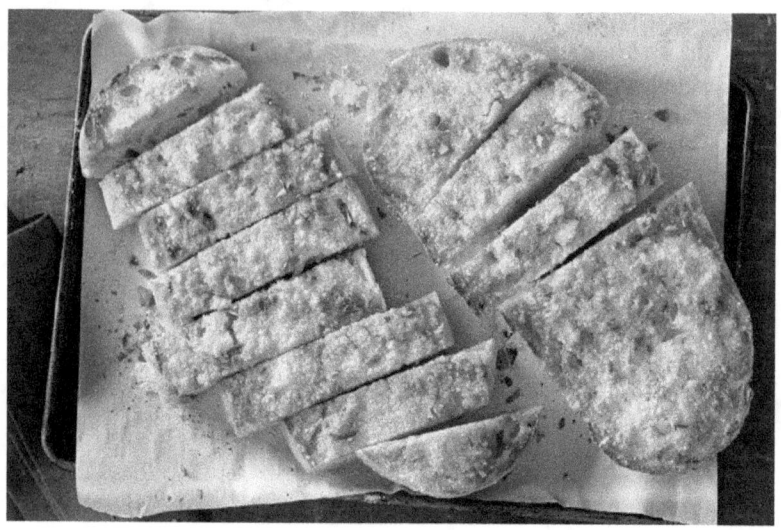

Anyone who has ever been on Keto or is tried the plan now will tell you that the most difficult meals to plan for are snacks. The breakfasts are straightforward, usually consisting of eggs, bacon, some other type of meat and veggies. Lunches are challenging, but if you don't mind making a large batch of one meal and freezing them, it is easy to make a quick lunch every day. Dinners are simple like breakfasts, meat, fat, and vegetables, repeat. If you are anything like me, you find that you get hungrier on Keto because your metabolism is speeding up. I find by the mid-morning (somewhere around 10:30) I am ravenous and I just want something quick and filling to quell the stomach pangs until lunchtime. I have found many different types of Keto snacks that are quick and easy to make and delicious to eat. Give some of these snacks a try the next time your stomach starts growling while following Keto.

1.Keto choco-nut balls

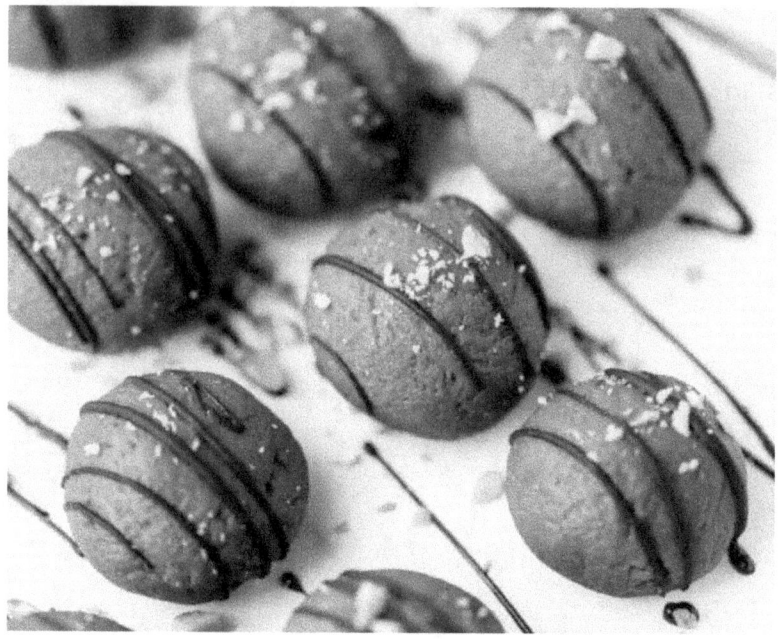

I love taking a few of these to work to snack on when hunger strikes. The taste is fabulous and it is even better after they have been in the freezer for a half hour or so.

Preparation Time-5 minutes

Servings-8

Ingredients

- 8 ounces softened cream cheese

- 4 ounces low-carb peanut butter
- 3 ounces coconut oil
- 1/2 teaspoon kosher salt
- 8 ounces dark chocolate chips

Directions

1. In a non-reactive bowl, mix all **Ingredients** except for chocolate chips and 1 ounce of coconut oil with a mixer until well combined. Place bowl in the freezer for 10-15 minutes.

2. Prepare a baking sheet by lining it with parchment paper and set aside. Remove the bowl from the freezer and scoop out dough with a spoon to make ping pong ball sized mounds. Transfer balls to the prepared baking sheet and place in the refrigerator for 5-10 minutes to harden.

3. In the meantime, mix chocolate chips and 1 ounce of coconut oil in a microwaveable bowl. Cook on high in 30-second intervals until fully melted.

4. Drizzle keto balls with the chocolate mixture and place back on the cookie sheet. Chill in the refrigerator for another 5-10 minutes before serving.

2.Bacon Guacamole balls

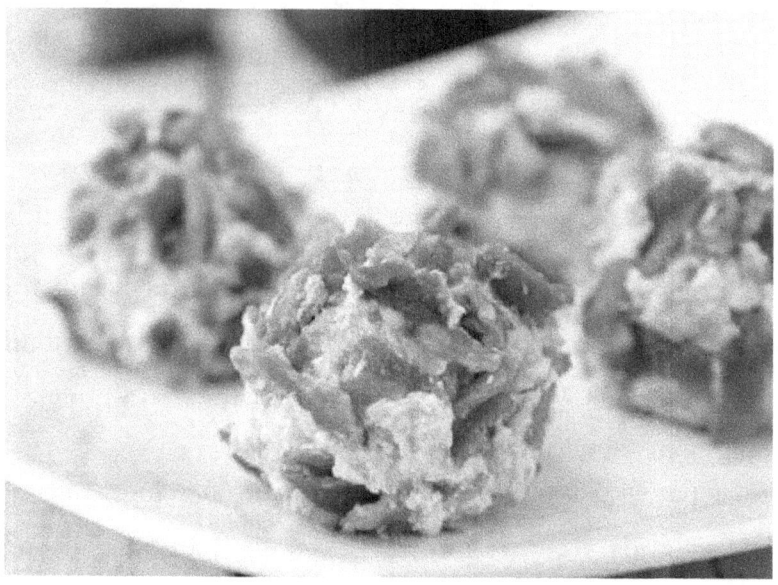

If you prefer a spicier dish, then leave the seeds in the jalapenos before chopping them. I use thick, fatty bacon for this recipe but you can also use chicken or turkey bacon if pork is a dietary restriction.

Preparation Time-10 minutes

Servings-15

Ingredients

- 10-12 slices cooked bacon, crumbled

GUACAMOLE

- 2 pitted and peeled avocados, mashed
- 6 ounces softened cream cheese
- 1 lime, juiced
- 1 minced clove garlic
- 1/4 minced red onion
- 1 seeded jalapeno, chopped
- 1 ounce chopped cilantro
- 1/2 teaspoon cumin
- 1/2 teaspoon chili powder
- Kosher salt
- Ground black pepper

Directions

1. Combine avocados, cream cheese, lime juice, garlic, onion, jalapeno, cilantro, cumin, chili, salt and pepper in a large mixing bowl. Stir until desired consistency is reached and chill in the refrigerator for 30-35 minutes.

Place bacon on a serving plate and scoop guacamole out of the bowl and into the bacon. Roll the guacamole in the bacon and transfer back to the plate. Chill in the refrigerator before serving.

3.Bacon Sushi

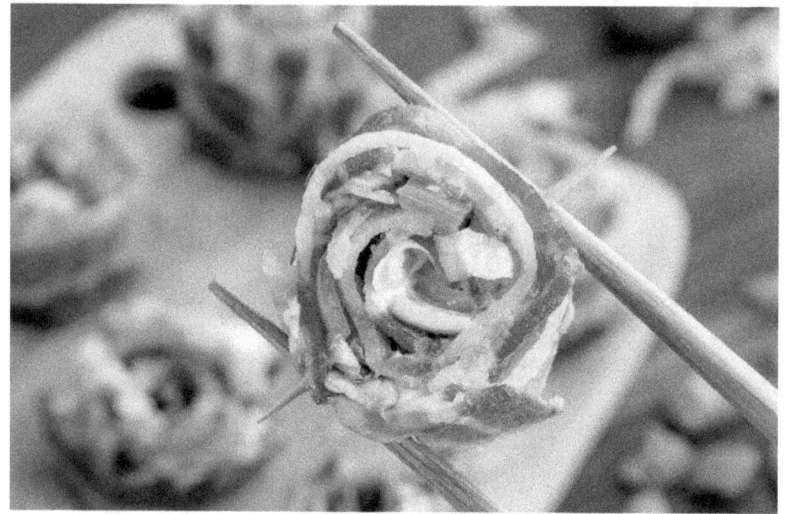

This bacon sushi hits the spot when the afternoon munchies strike. I like to use some 3-cheese Ranch dressing for dipping sauce.

Preparation Time-10 minutes

Servings-12

Ingredients

- 6 uncooked slices bacon, cut in half
- 2 thinly sliced Persian cucumbers
- 2 thinly sliced medium carrots

- 1 sliced avocado
- 4 ounces softened cream cheese
- Sesame seeds

Directions

1. Preheat oven to 400 degrees Fahrenheit

2. Line a cookie sheet with foil and place a baking on the sheet to allow cooling

3. Place bacon slices on the rack and cook for 10-15 minutes until desired crispiness is reached. The bacon should still be soft enough to manipulate.

4. Trim vegetables and avocado to the same width of the bacon.

5. Remove bacon and cool slightly. Spread cream cheese evenly on the bacon slices and dole out equal amounts of chopped veggies and avocado.

6. Roll bacon up into a spiral and secure with a toothpick.

7. Sprinkle with sesame seeds and enjoy!

4.Keto smoothie

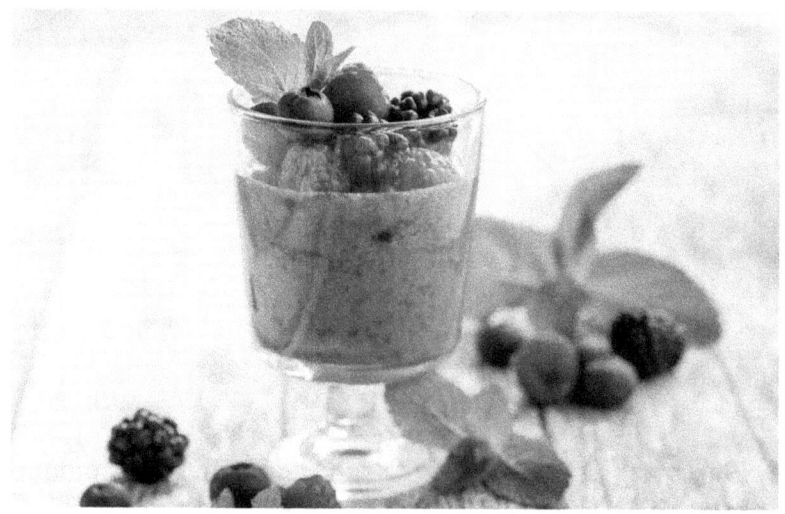

This delicious smoothie is shared with a friend or hoarded all for yourself! I like to top the smoothie off with some berries and coconut when I want a treat.

Preparation Time-5 minutes

Servings-2

Ingredients

- 16 ounces frozen raspberries
- 16 ounces frozen strawberries
- 16 ounces frozen blackberries

- 16 ounces coconut milk
- 8 ounces baby spinach
- 1/2 orange, juiced
- Shaved coconut, unsweetened

Directions

1. Place berries, milk, spinach, orange juice and coconut in a food processor and process until smooth.

2. Pour into cups and enjoy.

5.Keto tortillas

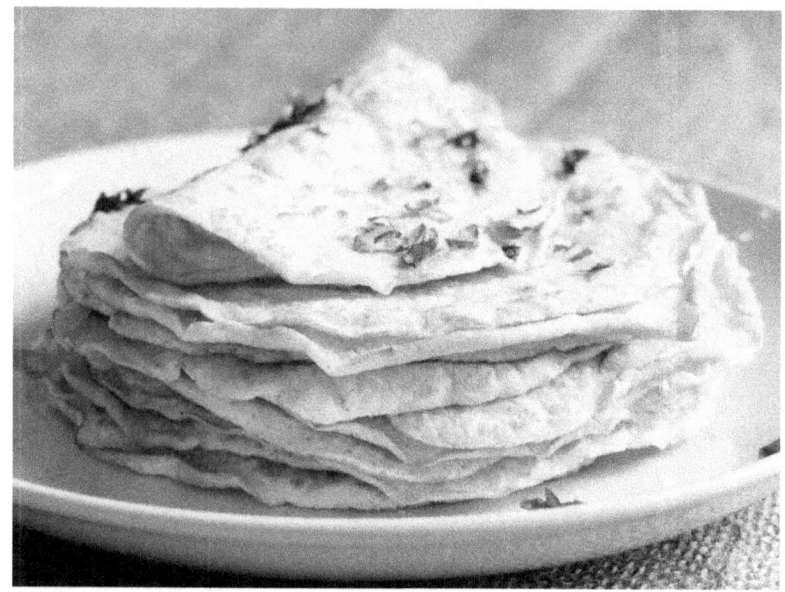

I bet you didn't think the word tortilla would be part of your Keto menu. This recipe is simple to make and satisfies the craving for carbohydrates that hits.

Preparation Time-20 minutes

Servings-8

Ingredients

- 8 ounces almond flour
- 2 ounces coconut flour

- 1/3 ounce xanthan gum

- 1/2 teaspoon kosher salt

- 1 teaspoon baking powder

- ½ ounce freshly squeezed lime juice

- 1 lightly beaten egg

- ½ ounce water

Directions

1. Place both flours, xanthan gum, Kosher salt and baking powder in a blender and process until combined.

2. Remove the top of the blender and while the motor is running, pour the last three **Ingredients** into the mixture and continue to process until it is a doughy consistency.

3. Remove dough from the blender and knead for 1-2 minutes. Wrap the ball in plastic and chill in the refrigerator for 10-15 minutes.

4. Split dough into 8 separate balls and wrap each one in 2 pieces of wax paper. Place wrapped balls on a flat surface and using a rolling pin, roll the dough to 1/8" thick. Unwrap tortillas from the wax paper.

5. Heat a large frying pan on medium high and cook tortillas for 20 seconds per side until slightly blackened.

6. Continue process until all tortillas are cooked and serve immediately with your favourite filling.

6.Bacon Cabbage Dippers

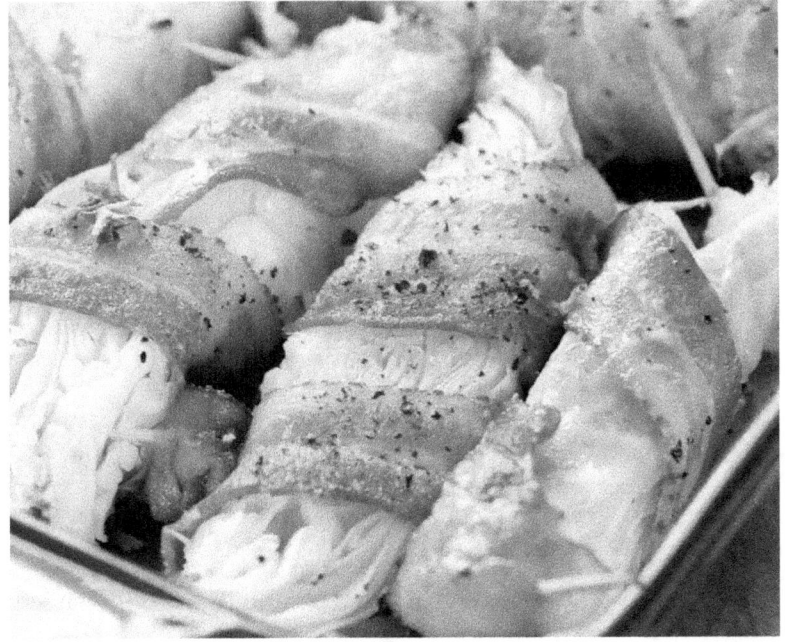

1. I like to serve these with some high-fat, low-carb Ranch-style dressing. The crispy texture of these dippers is addictive and will become your favourite go-to snack.

Preparation Time-15 minutes

Servings-8

Ingredients

- 1 medium head green cabbage, stemmed and quartered
- 2 ounces Parmesan cheese, grated
- 1 ounce extra-virgin olive oil
- 16 ounces bacon
- Kosher salt
- 1 teaspoon oregano, dried
- 1 teaspoon ground black pepper

Directions

2. Preheat oven to 450 degrees F. Coat the two baking sheets with a cooking spray.

3. Split each cabbage quarter in half and evenly divide between the two baking sheets.

4. Sprinkle the cabbage with parmesan and oil and toss gently to coat. Season with salt, oregano and black pepper.

5. Wrap each bacon slice around a wedge of cabbage and bake for 30 minutes until crispy and golden brown.

7.Chocolate Keto Protein Shake

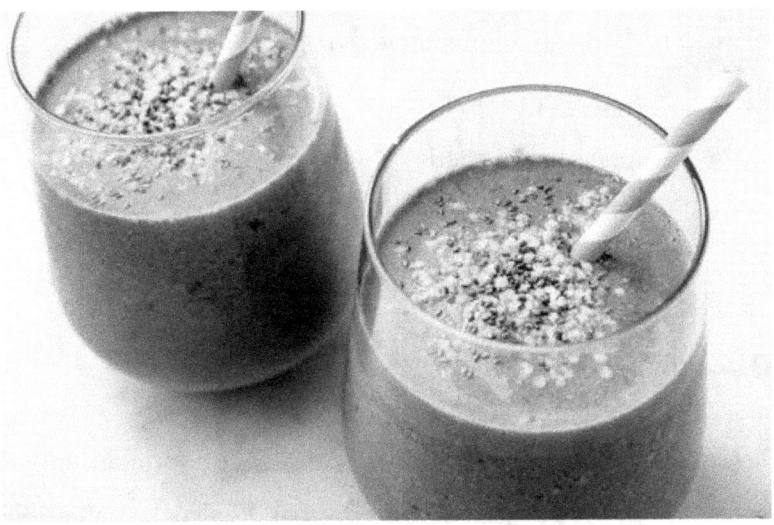

This shake will fill you up, give you energy and satisfy the Keto requirements of low-carb, high-fat foods. I like to make this shake in the morning when I'm in a hurry to get out of the door.

Preparation Time-5 minutes

Servings-1

Ingredients

- 6 ounces unsweetened almond milk
- 4 ounces crushed ice

- 1 ounce almond butter

- 1 ounce cocoa powder, unsweetened

- 1 ½ ounces Stevia sweetener

- ½ ounce chia seeds

- 1 ounce hemp seeds

- ¼ ounce vanilla extract

- 1 pinch kosher salt

Directions

1. Combine all the **Ingredients** in a blender and then blend until smooth. Next pour into a glass and garnish with some chia and hemp seeds.

8.Cucumber sushi

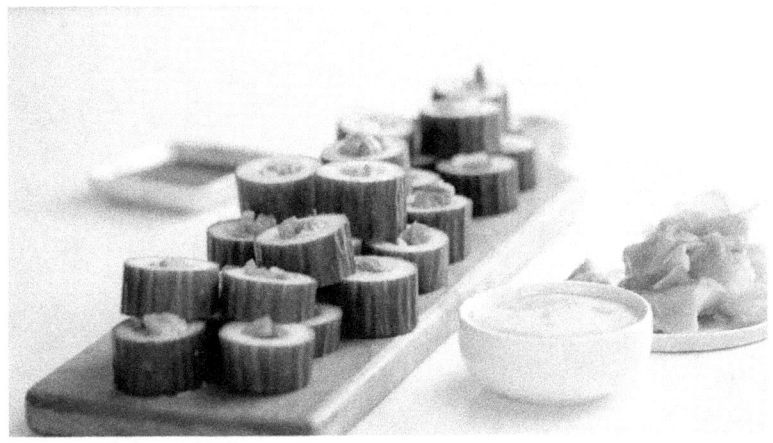

I love the sriracha with this cucumber sushi recipe. Why not make vegetables more interesting with some spicy dipping sauce?

Preparation Time-15 minutes

Servings-4

Ingredients

SUSHI

- 2 medium cucumbers, cut in half
- 1/4 thinly sliced avocado,
- 1/2 thinly sliced red bell pepper

- 1/2 thinly sliced yellow bell pepper
- 2 thinly sliced small carrots

DIPPING SAUCE

- 1 teaspoon soy sauce
- ½ ounce sriracha sauce
- 2 ½ ounces mayonnaise

Directions

1. Scoop seeds and pulp from cucumber halves until they are hollowed out.

2. Place sliced avocado in the middle of the cucumber and press down until evenly filled.

3. Add peppers and carrots to the avocado in the cucumber until full

4. Slice cucumber into 1" slices

5. Make the sauce by combining the dipping sauce Ingredients and serve with the sliced cucumber sushi.

9.Keto Cereal

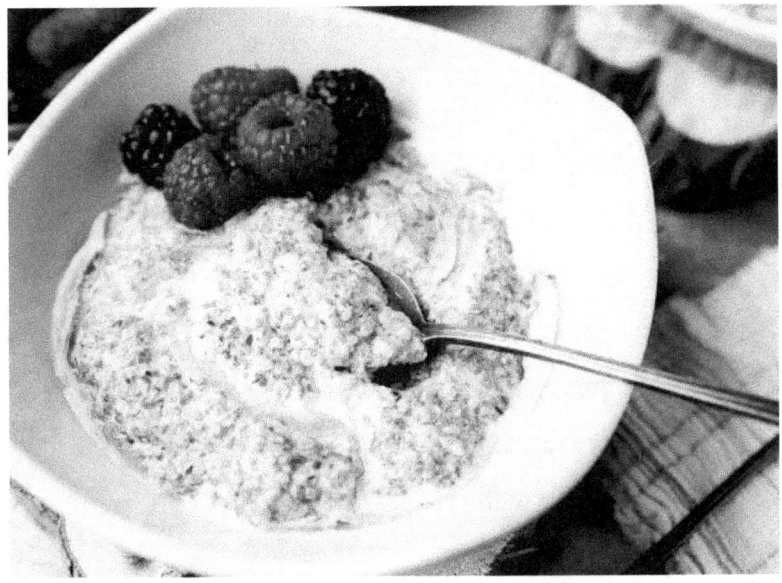

Cereal is not a word normally associated with Keto, but this recipe will satisfy the carb-lover in you! I like to make this in the morning and pack some for a snack for the afternoon.

Preparation Time-10 minutes

Servings-24 ounces

Ingredients

- Cooking spray
- 8 ounces chopped almonds

- 8 ounces chopped walnuts
- 2 ounces sesame seeds
- 8 ounces coconut flakes, unsweetened
- 1 ounce chia seeds
- 1 ounce flax seeds
- 1/2 teaspoon clove, ground
- 1/2 teaspoon kosher salt
- ¼ ounce ground cinnamon
- 1 teaspoon vanilla extract
- 2 ounces coconut oil, melted
- 1 large egg white

Directions

1. Preheat oven to 350 degrees F. Coat a baking sheet with a cooking spray and set aside.

2. Combine nuts, coconut and seeds in a large mixing bowl. Add cinnamon, salt, cloves and vanilla and stir well.

3. In a separate bowl, beat the egg whites until frothy and add to the seeds and nuts mixture. Stir until coated. Stir in coconut oil and pour into the baking sheet.

4. Bake for 20-25 minutes until golden, stirring after 15 minutes.

5. Cool and serve.

10.Jalapeno popper egg cups

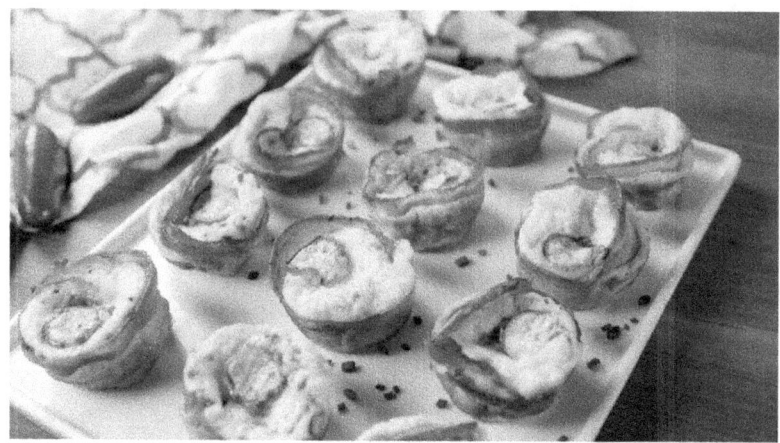

You will find that you eat a lot of eggs on Keto. It can get monotonous unless you spice up your recipes and try something new like these egg cups.

Preparation Time-10 minutes

Servings-12

Ingredients

- 12 uncooked bacon slices
- 10 eggs
- 2 ounces sour cream
- 4 ounces Cheddar cheese, shredded
- 1 teaspoon garlic powder

- 4 ounces mozzarella cheese, shredded
- 1 minced jalapeño pepper
- 1 thinly sliced jalapeño pepper
- kosher salt
- Freshly ground black pepper
- nonstick cooking spray

Directions

1. Preheat oven to 375 degrees Fahrenheit. Coat a 12-cup muffin tin with a cooking spray.

2. Cook bacon in a large frying pan on Medium until it is cooked but not crispy. Then remove the bacon and drain on a paper towel.

3. Whisk eggs, sour cream, jalapeno and garlic powder in a large mixing bowl until well combined. Sprinkle with salt and pepper to taste.

4. Line a muffin cup with 1 piece of bacon and pour the egg mixture over, leaving 1/3 of space at the top of the cup. Top with jalapeno and bake for 20-25 minutes until eggs are set.

11.Hard Boiled Eggs

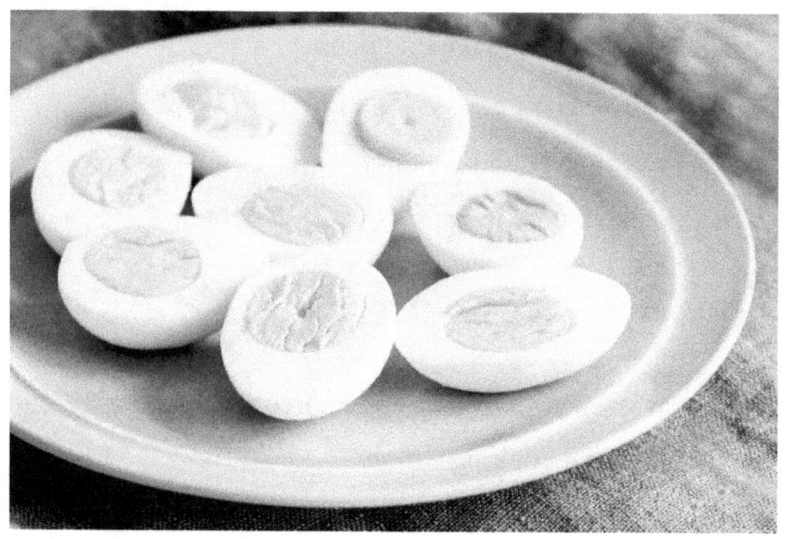

There's nothing wrong with going the traditional way and cooking up some hard-boiled eggs. I like to eat them with a generous portion of full-fat mayonnaise and a little bit of salt.

Preparation Time-5 minutes

Servings-12

Ingredients

- 12 large eggs
- water

Directions

1. Bring a large pot of water to boil and delicately place eggs in the boiling water with a slotted spoon. Set the timer for 12 minutes and when time is up, drain eggs in a colander. Pour the cold water over the eggs and when they are cool enough to handle, peel them.

12.Carrot cake keto balls

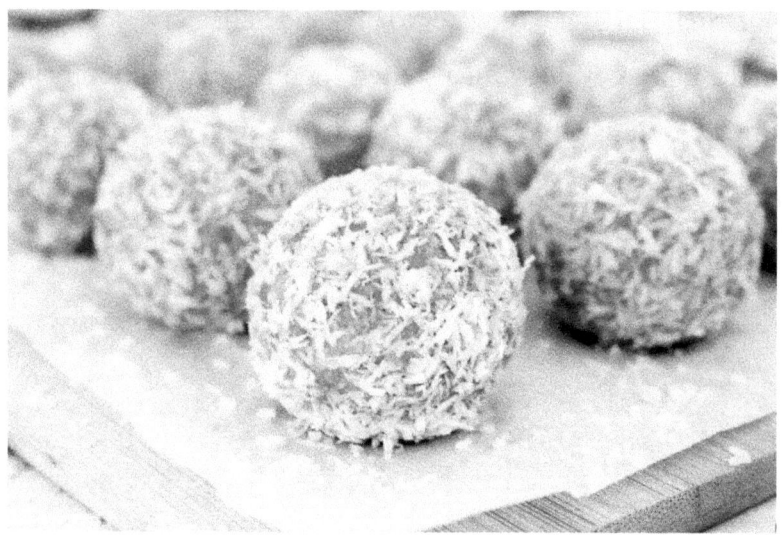

Cake on the Keto diet? This recipe brings the delicious sweetness of dessert without all the pesky carbs.

Preparation Time-5 minutes

Servings-16

Ingredients

- 8 ounces softened cream cheese
- 6 ounces coconut flour
- 1 teaspoon stevia granules or another sweetener
- ½ teaspoon vanilla extract

- 1 teaspoon cinnamon
- ¼ teaspoon nutmeg, ground
- 8 ounces carrots, grated
- 4 ounces pecans, chopped
- 8 ounces unsweetened coconut, shredded

Directions

1. Beat cream cheese, flour, sweetener, vanilla extract, cinnamon and nutmeg in a large mixing bowl until smooth and creamy. Fold nuts and carrots into the batter until just combined.

2. Form batter into golf-ball shaped mounds and roll them in the coconut. Chill for 10 minutes and serve

13.Keto bread

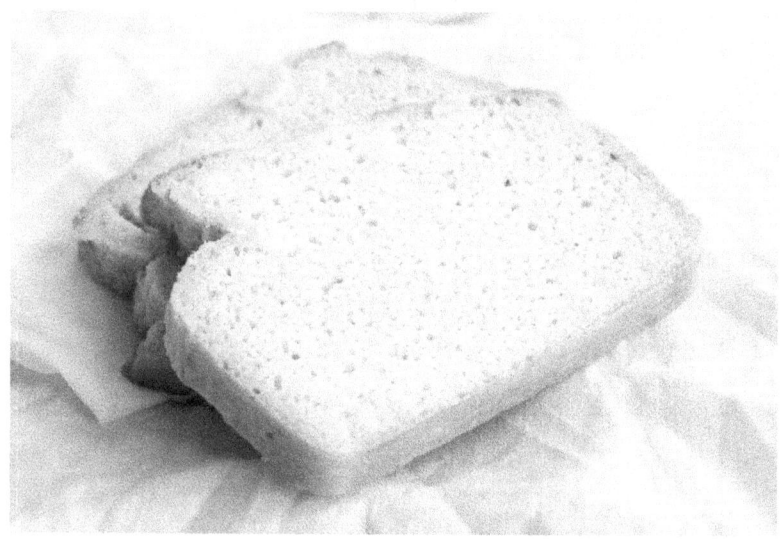

Keto bread may seem like a typo, but this recipe satisfies the need for bread without all the carbs. This bread is delicious spread with some cream cheese and tomato slices in the morning.

Preparation Time-10 minutes

Servings-1

Ingredients

- 6 large eggs, whites and yolks separated
- 1/2 teaspoon cream of tartar

- 2 ounces melted butter, cooled
- 12 ounces almond flour, finely ground
- ½ ounce baking powder
- 1/2 teaspoon kosher salt

Directions

1. Preheat oven to 375 degrees Fahrenheit. Line a 5x9 loaf pan with parchment and set aside.

2. Beat egg whites and cream of tartar in a large mixing bowl with a manual mixer until you see peaks forming.

3. Beat yolks and butter in another large mixing bowl with a manual mixer. Add almond flour, salt and baking powder to the yolk mixture and beat until well combined.

4. Fold in a third of the egg white mixture to the egg yolk mix until combined. Fold in the other 2/3 of egg whites and pour into prepared loaf pan.

5. Bake for about 30 minutes until a tester put in the middle has come out clean. Cool before serving.

14.Keto Brownie Balls

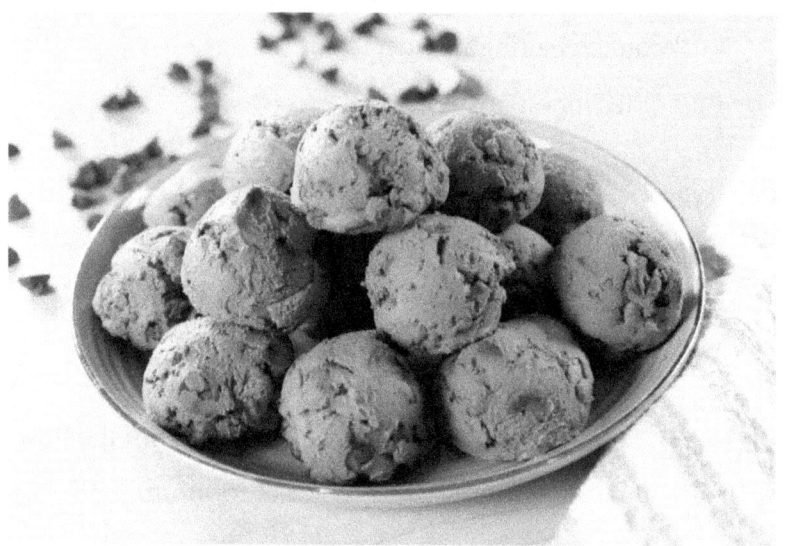

My kids love stealing these brownie balls for their lunches and snacks so I always have to make triple the amount so I have some for myself. I like to eat them slightly frozen as they are delicious!

Preparation Time-15 minutes

Servings-5

Ingredients

- 8 ounces softened cream cheese
- 2 ounces coconut oil

- 2 ounces cocoa powder, unsweetened
- 5 ½ ounces dark chocolate chips

Directions

1. Line a baking sheet with parchment paper.

2. Beat all **Ingredients** together in a large mixing bowl except for chocolate chips until well combined. Fold in chips until a dough forms.

3. Scoop small balls onto the cookie sheet and freeze for 20 minutes before serving.

15.Keto taquitos

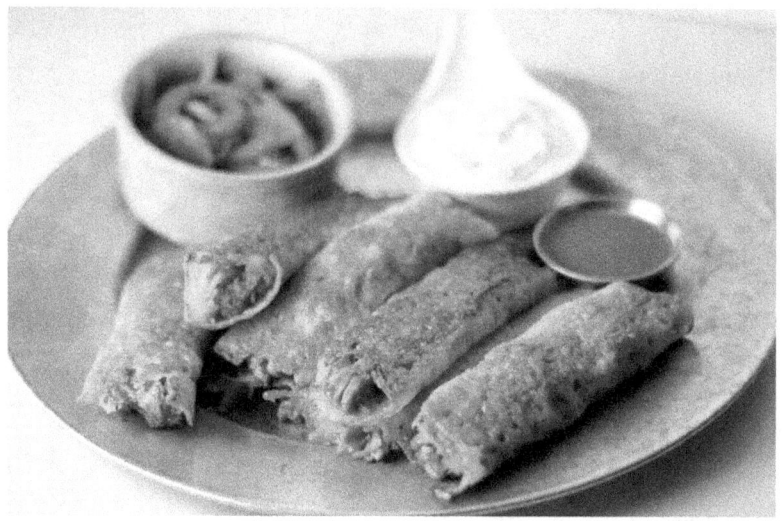

This dish is not just fun to say but amazing to eat! I will make these on the weekend when I don't have too much to do and I want to enjoy a leisurely lunch.

Preparation Time-15 minutes

Servings-6

Ingredients

- ½ ounce extra-virgin olive oil
- 1/4 finely chopped onion
- 2 minced garlic cloves

- 1/2 teaspoon cumin
- 1/2 teaspoon chili powder
- 12 ounces cooked chicken, shredded
- 2 ½ ounces red enchilada sauce
- 1 ounce cilantro, chopped
- Kosher salt
- 8 ounces Cheddar cheese, shredded
- 8 ounces Monterey Jack cheese, shredded
- Sour cream

Directions

1. Preheat oven to 375 degrees Fahrenheit. Line a baking sheet with parchment and set aside.

2. Heat oil in a frying pan on Medium heat. Sautee onion in the oil for three minutes until softened. Stir in the cumin, chile powder and garlic and cook for another minute or two until fragrant.

3. Stir in chicken and enchilada sauce and bring to a simmer. Add cilantro and salt, stir and remove pan from heat.

4. For taquito shells-

5. Combine Cheddar and Monterey jack cheeses in a large mixing bowl. Evenly divide cheese mix in six flat mounds on the baking sheet. Bake for 8-10 minutes until cheese is melted and golden brown on the edges, but still pliable.

6. Remove cheese from the oven and cool for 2-4 minutes. Add chicken mixture to the cheese mounds and roll the filling up tight.

7. Serve with sour cream and top with extra cilantro.

16.Keto Garlic Bread

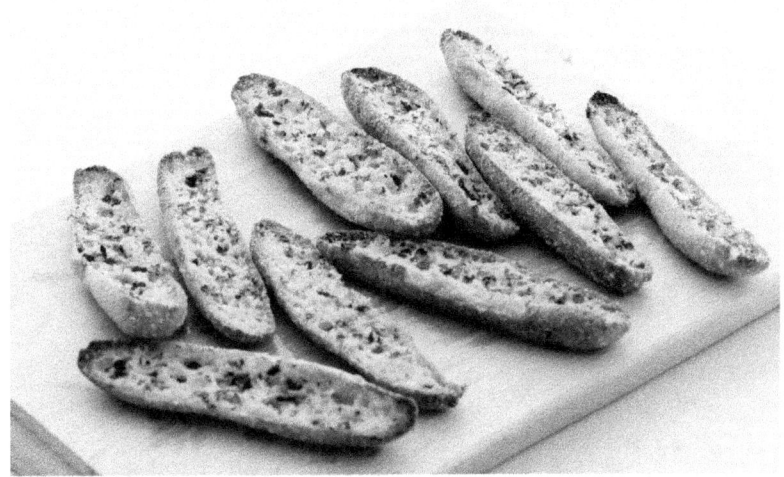

Slice and serve with warmed marinara sauce for dipping or some salsa and sour cream. This garlic 'bread' makes a delicious side dish for a filling Keto dinner.

Preparation Time-5 minutes

Servings-4

Ingredients

- 8 ounces mozzarella cheese, shredded
- 4 ounces almond flour
- 1 ounce softened cream cheese

- ½ ounce garlic powder

- 1 teaspoon baking powder

- Kosher salt

- 1 large egg

- ½ ounce melted butter

- 1 minced clove garlic

- ½ ounce parsley, chopped

- ½ ounce Parmesan cheese, grated

Directions

1. Preheat oven to 400 degrees Fahrenheit. Line a medium baking sheet with parchment and set aside.

2. In a large microwaveable bowl, combine mozzarella cheese, flour, cream cheese, garlic, baking powder and Kosher salt. Stir well and cook on High for 1 minute until cheese is melted.

3. Remove bowl and crack an egg into the mixture. Stir until a dough forms.

4. Place dough on the baking sheet and shape into an oval of ½" thickness.

5. Combine the rest of the **Ingredients** in a small separate bowl and brush over the surface of the dough.

6. Bake for 15-17 minutes until golden brown on top. Cool slightly before serving.

17.Avocado Crab Boats

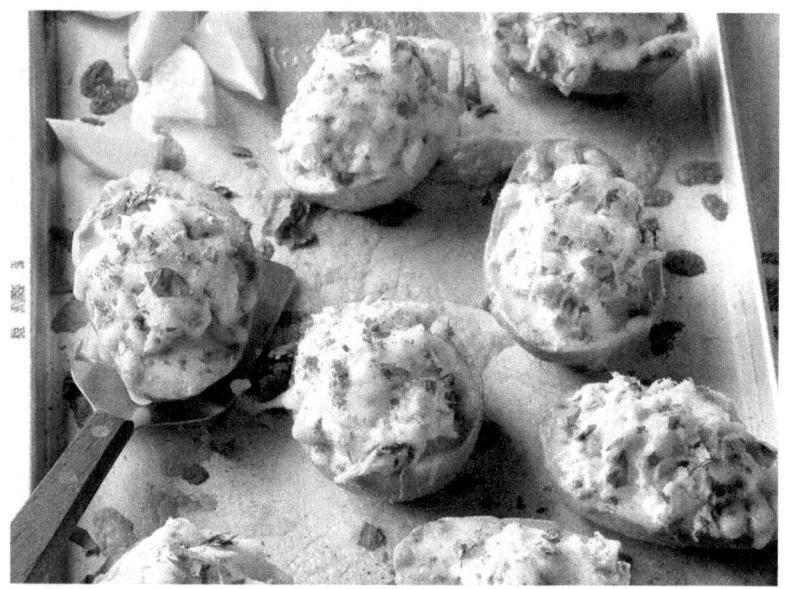

These delicious and colourful treats are the perfect appetizer for you and your fellow Keto-followers. I like to put the avocado in the fridge for a few minutes so it is easier to work with.

Preparation Time-5 minutes

Servings-4

Ingredients

- 12 ounces lump crab meat

- 2 ½ ounces plain Greek yogurt

- 1/2 minced red onion

- 1 ounce chives, Chopped

- 1 ½ ounces lemon juice

- 1/2 teaspoon cayenne pepper

- kosher salt

- 8 ounces Cheddar cheese, shredded

- 2 avocados, cut in half with stones removed

Directions

1. Stir together all **Ingredients** except for avocados and cheddar cheese in a mixing bowl until well combined.

2. Scoop some of the avocado, leaving enough avocado around the border to create a small bowl out of the fruit. Dice the avocado you scooped out and incorporate it into the crab mix.

3. Preheat broiler and place avocado bowls on a baking sheet. Broil for 1 minute and serve right away.

18.Ham and Cheese egg cups

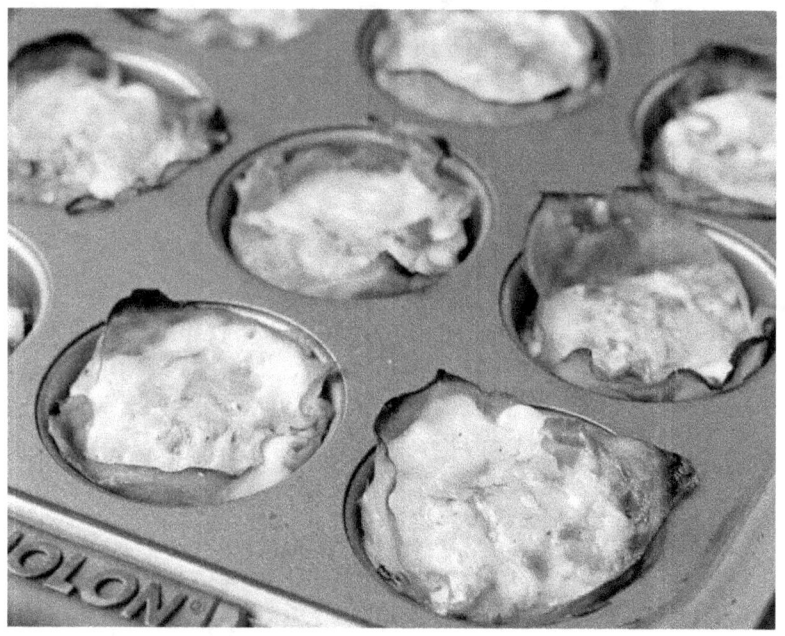

This recipe is perfect when you are looking for new and interesting lunch and breakfast ideas. I like to make a batch of these in the evening so I have enough for a few days.

Preparation Time-5 minutes

Servings-12

Ingredients

- Cooking spray, for pan

- 12 slices deli ham
- 8 ounces cheddar cheese, shredded
- 12 eggs
- kosher salt
- black pepper
- Parsley, chopped

Directions

1. Preheat oven to 400 degrees Fahrenheit. Line a 12-cup muffin tin with paper liners. Add a slice of ham and a small portion of cheddar cheese to each cup. Then crack an egg into the cup and sprinkle with salt and pepper.

2. Bake for 12-15 minutes until eggs are set to your liking.

3. Top with parsley and enjoy!

19.Creamy avocado dip

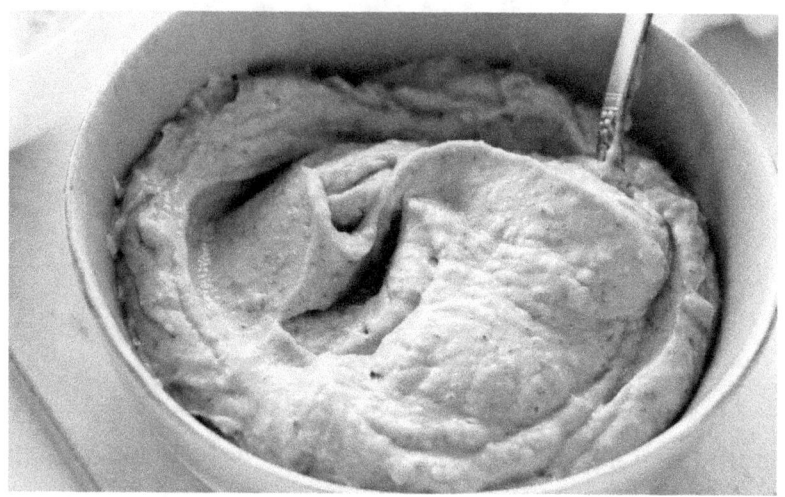

I like to serve this dip with some cauliflower florets and carrot sticks. It also tastes amazing spread over some chicken with 3-cheese Ranch dressing and shredded cheese.

Preparation Time-5 minutes

Servings-4

Ingredients

- 2 ripened peeled and pitted avocados, mashed
- 4 ounces plain Greek yogurt
- 2 minced garlic cloves
- 1 lime, juiced

- Kosher salt
- black pepper

Directions

1. Combine all Ingredients together in a serving bowl and enjoy!

20.Ham, egg and cheese roll-ups

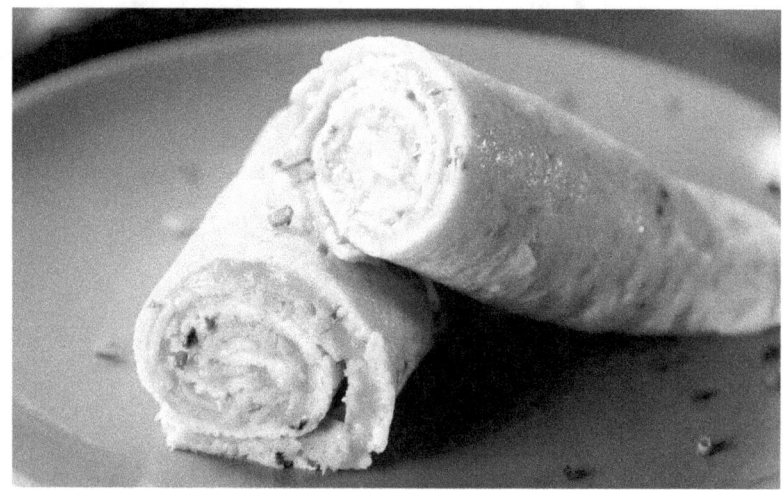

These roll-ups are perfect for when you want to load up on fat and protein before leaving for work. They will keep you full and are simple to make for any meal.

Preparation Time-20 minutes

Servings-5

Ingredients

- 10 large eggs
- 1/3 ounce garlic powder
- kosher salt
- black pepper

- 1 ounce butter
- 12 ounces Cheddar Cheese, shredded
- 8 ounces baby spinach
- 8 ounces tomatoes, chopped
- 20 slices deli ham

Directions

1. Pre-heat the oven's broiler. Lightly spray a shallow baking dish and set aside.

2. Whisk eggs, cheese, garlic, salt and pepper together in a large mixing bowl.

3. Melt butter in a frying pan on medium heat and pour egg mixture into the pan. Cook eggs in pan for 3 minutes, stirring occasionally until cheese melts. Add spinach and tomatoes to the mixture in the pan and stir until well combined.

4. Arrange two slices of ham on a serving dish and top with eggs. Roll the ham and place in the baking dish. Repeat with the other slices of ham and broil in the oven for 5 minutes until crispy.

21.Bacon avocado balls

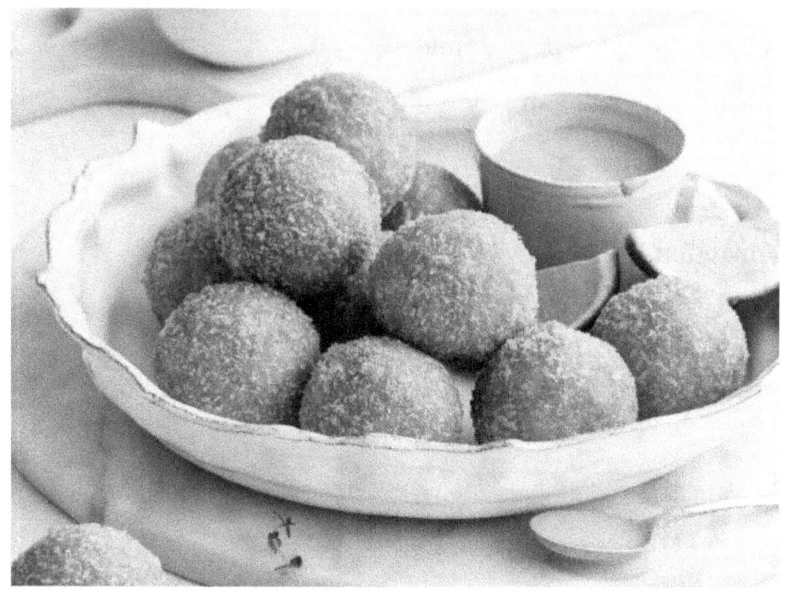

The smoky flavor of the bacon tastes amazing when mixed with the cheese and avocado. This recipe tastes best hot from the oven.

Preparation Time-10 minutes

Servings-4

Ingredients

- 2 ripened avocados, peeled, pitted and halved
- 2 ½ ounces Cheddar cheese, shredded

- 8 uncooked slices bacon

Directions

1. Preheat broiler. Line a baking sheet with a parchment or an aluminum foil and set aside.

2. Fill two avocado halves with cheddar cheese and place the other half on top to close it. Wrap the two halves with 4 pieces of bacon.

3. Place on the baking sheet and then bake for 5 minutes under the broiler until crispy on the top. Flip the avocados over and broil for another 5 minutes.

4. Cut in half and serve.

22.Turkey club cups

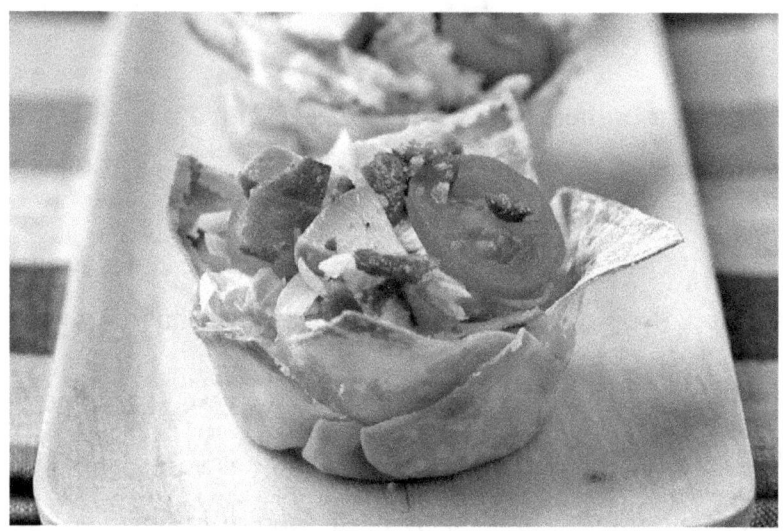

These turkey cups make an ideal treat when you get the munchies in the middle of the day. You can bring a couple to work and enjoy them for a mid-morning snack as well.

Preparation Time-10 minutes

Servings-14

Ingredients

- 14 slices sharp cheddar
- 14 slices roasted deli turkey
- 2 ounces full-fat mayonnaise

- 1 ounce Dijon mustard

- 1/2 shredded head iceberg lettuce

- 16 ounces chopped cherry tomatoes

- 1 peeled, pitted and chopped avocado

- 8 cooked slices bacon, crumbled

Directions

1. Preheat oven to 400 degrees Fahrenheit. Coat a 12-cup muffin tin with a cooking spray or line with paper liners.

2. Arrange a slice of turkey in each cup and add a slice of cheddar. Bake for 10 minutes until cheese is melted.

3. Mix mayonnaise and mustard in a small bowl and add a spoonful to each muffin cup. Fill each with even amounts of the rest of the **Ingredients** and enjoy!

23.Brussels sprout chips

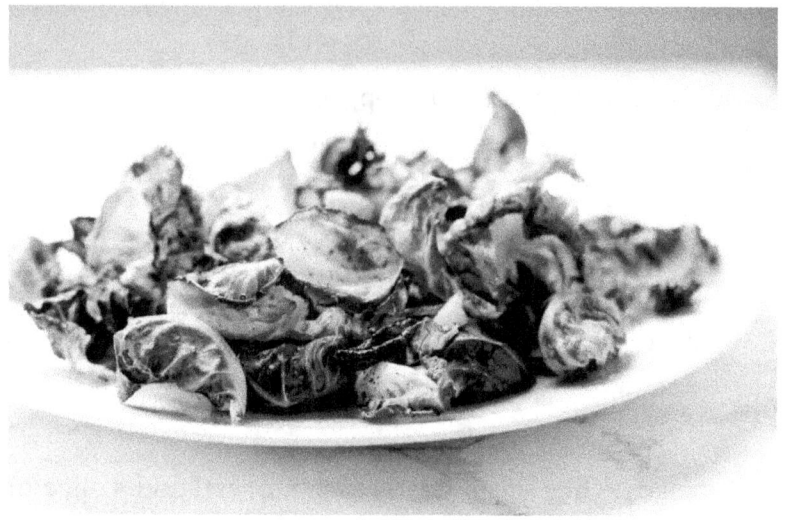

When you are craving a crunchy chip taste, give these Keto-friendly treats a try! The Kosher salt has a stronger taste than table salt, so go easy on it if you don't like your food too salty.

Preparation Time-5 minutes

Servings-2-3

Ingredients

- 1 teaspoon of garlic powder
- 8 Brussels sprouts, thinly sliced

- ½ ounce extra-virgin olive oil

- 1 ounce Parmesan cheese, grated

- Kosher salt

- black pepper

- High fat low-carb Caesar salad dressing

Directions

1. Preheat oven to 400 degrees F. Lightly coat a medium baking sheet with a cooking spray.

Mix oil, cheese and garlic powder in a large mixing bowl with salt and pepper. Toss sprouts in the mixture until coated.

Arrange Brussels sprouts on the prepared baking sheet and bake for 10 minutes. Toss the sprouts and bake for another 10 minutes until golden and crispy.

Top with extra Parmesan and Caesar dressing for dipping.

24.No-bread subs

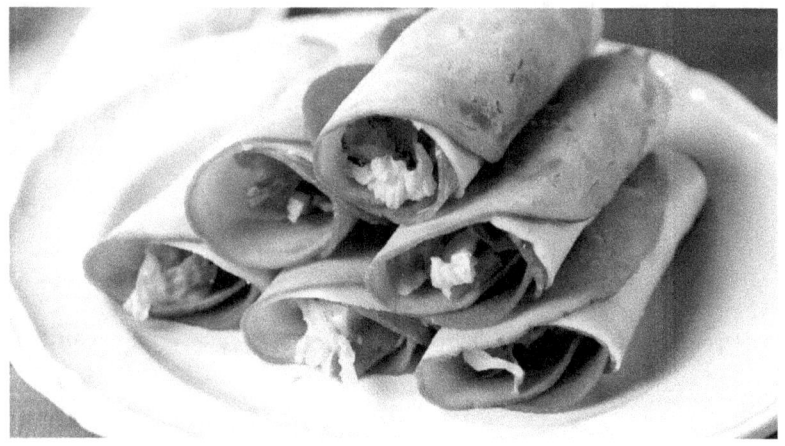

These subs taste amazing and you won't even notice the bread is gone. I like to try different combinations of **Ingredients** for variety throughout the week.

Preparation Time-15 minutes

Servings-6

Ingredients

- 4 ounces high-fat mayonnaise
- 1 ounce red wine vinegar
- ½ ounce extra-virgin olive oil
- 1 small grated garlic clove
- 1 teaspoon Italian seasoning

- 12 slices pepperoni
- 6 slices deli ham
- 6 slices provolone
- 12 slices salami
- 8 ounces romaine lettuce, shredded
- 4 ounces red peppers, roasted

Directions

1. On a serving plate, layer your sandwich in the following way – 1 slice of ham, 2 slices of salami, 2 slices of pepperoni and 1 slice of provolone cheese.

2. Whisk mayonnaise, vinegar, garlic, oil and seasoning together in a small bowl.

3. Add some romaine and red peppers in the middle of the sandwich and drizzle with mayonnaise mixture.

4. Roll up your sub and enjoy. You should have enough for 6.

25.Chicken bacon ranch poppers

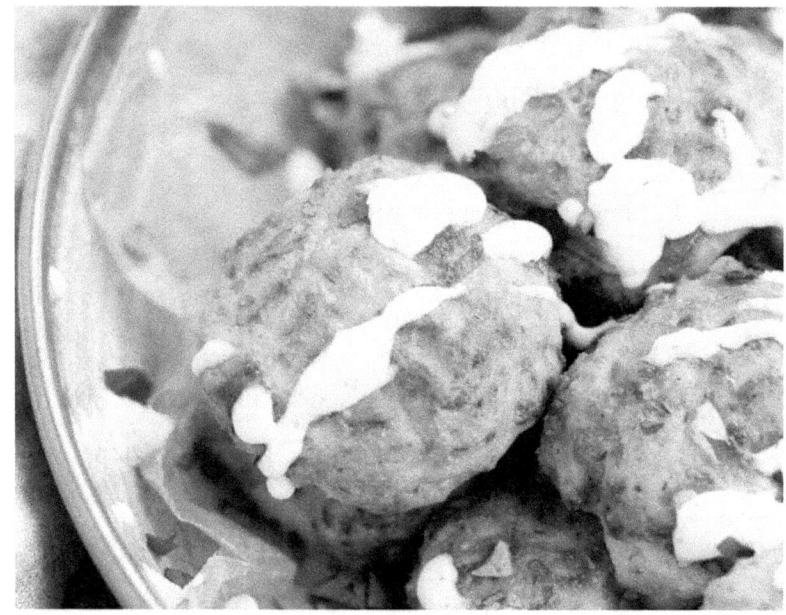

I like to make these for movie night and stuff my face as I watch my favourite show. These taste amazing with ranch or blue cheese dressing for dipping.

Preparation Time-5 minutes

Servings-15

Ingredients

- 16 ounces ground chicken
- 6 cooked slices bacon, crumbled

- 1 large beaten egg
- ½ ounce high-fat ranch seasoning
- Kosher salt
- black pepper

Directions

1. Preheat oven to 375 degrees Fahrenheit. Coat a baking sheet with a cooking spray.

2. Combine all Ingredients in a large mixing bowl.

3. Form into golf-ball sized balls and place on baking sheet. Flatten to desired width and bake for 30 minutes until cooked through.

26.Cookie dough keto balls

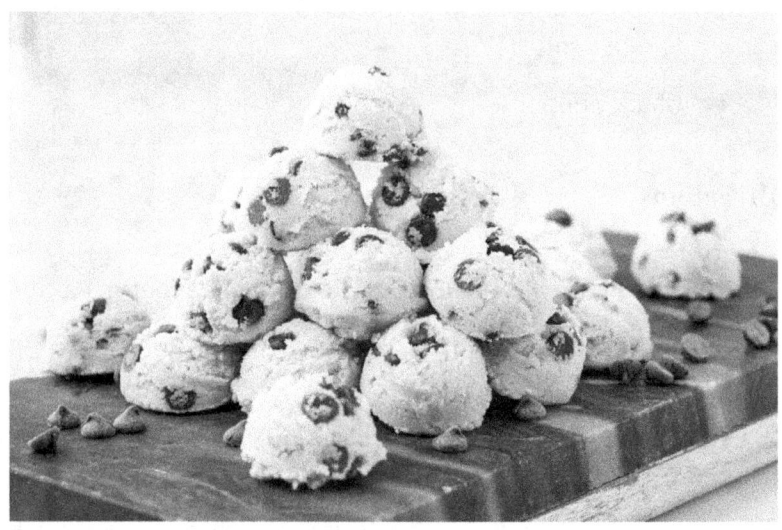

I usually use Lily's chocolate for any of my Keto recipes. This dark chocolate has a low carb count and uses Stevia for sweetener instead of sugar.

Preparation Time-5 minutes

Servings-15

Ingredients

- 4 ounces softened butter
- 2 ½ ounces Swerve confectioners' sugar
- 1/2 teaspoon vanilla extract

- 1/2 teaspoon kosher salt
- 16 ounces almond flour
- 5 ½ ounces dark chocolate chips

Directions

1. Beat butter in a large mixing bowl with an electric mixer until creamy and fluffy.

2. Beat in Swerve, vanilla extract and salt until well combined.

3. Gradually beat in flour until moistened and fold the chocolate into the batter.

4. Wrap the bowl in plastic and chill in the refrigerator for 15-20 minutes until slightly firm.

5. Remove bowl from the refrigerator and scoop dough balls out with a tablespoon.

6. Transfer dough balls to a large plastic container and store in the refrigerator.

27.Bacon Asparagus Bites

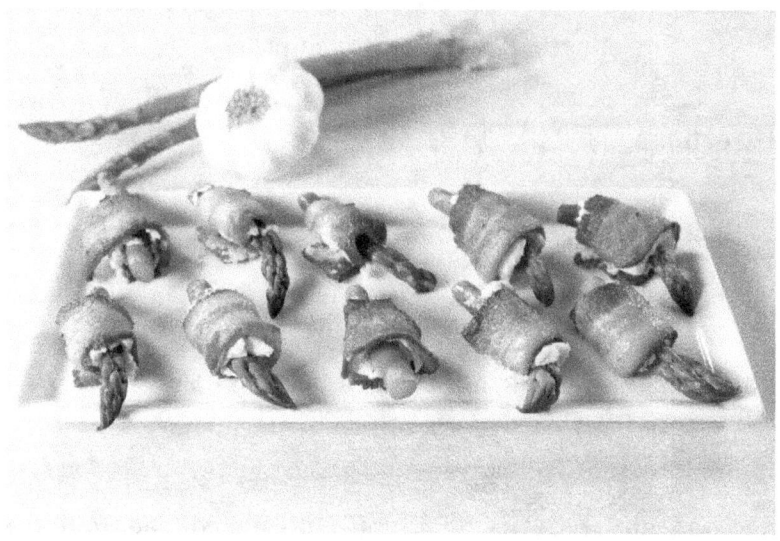

I love the taste of bacon and asparagus and this recipe is one of my favourites to make. I like to have these on hand when I am watching television or while playing games with my kids.

Preparation Time-10 minutes

Servings-6

Ingredients

- 6 slices bacon, sliced into thirds
- 5 ounces softened cream cheese

- 1 minced garlic clove
- Kosher salt
- Ground black pepper
- 9 blanched and trimmed asparagus spears

Directions

1. Preheat oven to 400 degrees Fahrenheit. Line a baking sheet with parchment.

2. Cook bacon in a large frying pan on medium heat until bacon is browned but not crispy. Drain bacon on a paper towel.

3. Mix cream cheese, garlic, salt and pepper in a small bowl until well combined.

4. Arrange bacon on the baking sheet. Spread ¼ ounce of cream cheese mixture on each strip.

5. Place a spear of asparagus in the center of the cream cheese and roll the bacon tightly. Repeat process for each bacon roll.

6. Bake for 5 minutes until bacon is crispy.

28. Keto Jalapeno Popper bread

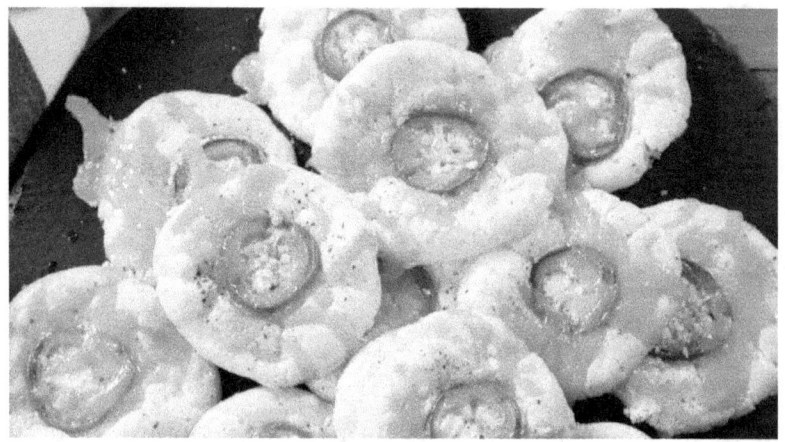

This bread is delicious to make at any time, not just when you are on Keto. My family always takes half of these poppers for themselves so I like to bake a few batches at a time.

Preparation Time-15 minutes

Servings-16

Ingredients

- 3/4 teaspoon cream of tartar
- 6 egg whites
- 4 egg yolks
- 2 ounces softened cream cheese

- 1 teaspoon garlic powder
- 3/4 teaspoon kosher salt
- 4 ounces cheddar cheese, shredded
- 1 thinly sliced jalapeño

Directions

1. Preheat oven to 300 degrees Fahrenheit. Coat a medium baking sheet with a cooking spray.

2. Whisk egg whites with cream of tartar in a large mixing bowl until you see peaks forming.

3. In another bowl, beat cream cheese, yolks, garlic and salt until well combined. Fold egg white mixture and cheddar cheese into the cream cheese mixture.

4. Place 2 ounce scoops onto the baking sheet and top with jalapeno.

5. Bake for 25-30 minutes until puffy and golden brown.

29.Smoked salmon pâté with cucumber

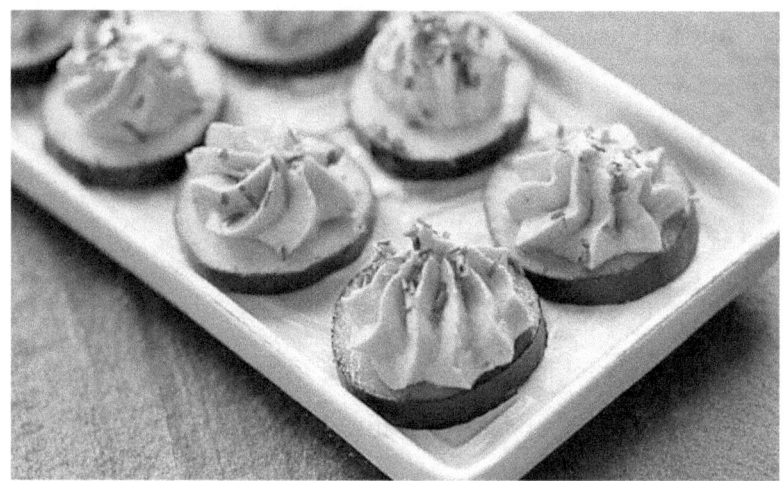

Smoked salmon is one of my favourite foods while on Keto. This salmon pâté recipe is simple to make and taste delicious with everything, from vegetables to meat.

Preparation Time-15 minutes

Servings-12

Ingredients

- 4 ½ ounces smoked salmon
- 5 ½ ounces softened cream cheese
- 2 ounces heavy cream

- ½ ounce freshly squeezed lemon juice
- ½ ounce fresh chives
- Kosher salt
- Ground black pepper
- 2 Cucumbers, peeled and sliced into 2" slices

Directions

1. Scoop out the fleshy part of the cucumber using a spoon but leave some flesh near the bottom of the slice to make a cup.

2. Combine ¾ of smoked salmon, cream cheese, cream, salt, lemon juice, chives and pepper in a blender and process until smooth.

3. Chop up the rest of the salmon and add to the pate.

4. Fill each cucumber cup with some pate and enjoy!

30.Curry chicken lettuce wraps

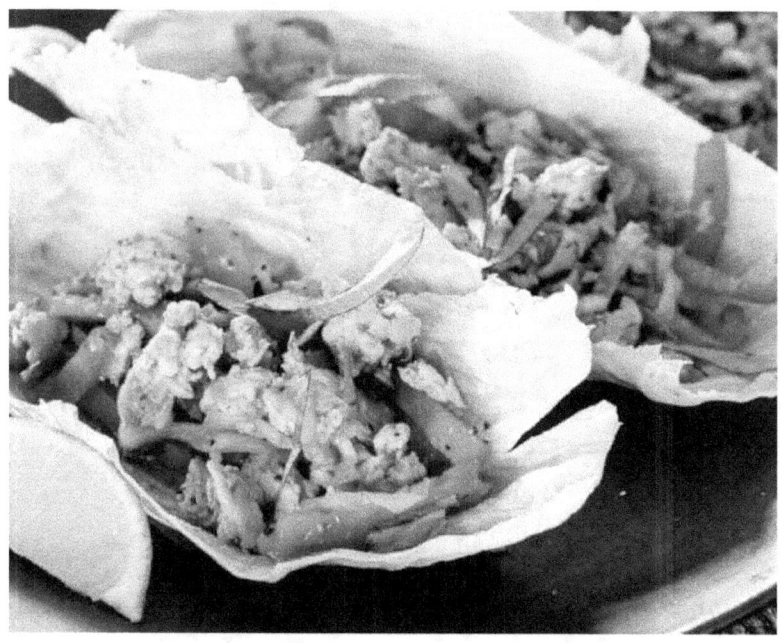

I love the flavor of these delectable lettuce wraps and they make an ideal late night snack. Try them with some sour cream or plain Greek yogurt.

Preparation Time-15 minutes

Servings-2

Ingredients

- 16 ounces skinless and boneless chicken thighs, cut in 1" pieces
- 2 ounces onion, minced
- 2 garlic cloves, minced
- 1/3 ounce Curry Powder
- ¼ ounce pink Himalayan salt
- 1 teaspoon ground black pepper
- 1 ½ ounces ghee
- 8 ounces cauliflower rice
- 6-8 small lettuce leaves
- 2 ounces plain coconut milk yogurt, unsweetened

INSTRUCTIONS

1. Heat a big frying pan on medium heat. Add 1 ounce of ghee and onion and sauté until browned.

2. Stir in chicken pieces, garlic and salt for 8 minutes until chicken is browned and no longer pink in the middle.

3. Stir in the rest of the ghee, curry and rice and cook until well combined and heated through.

4. Arrange lettuce leaves on a serving plate and scoop out chicken mixture onto the leaves.

5. Top with coconut yogurt and enjoy!

Conclusion

Whether you are new at Keto or familiar with the meal plan, you can agree that snacks are especially challenging. This cookbook is meant as a guide for those people who don't have a lot of time to prepare food, but want the health benefits a Keto diet provides. These 30 snacks are quick and easy, taste great and will keep you in a state of ketosis because they are high in fat and low in carbohydrates. Gives them a try today for the next time you feel like a quick snack throughout the day.